Staying HEALTHY with dr. nature

An Essential Oils Cookbook and Aromatherapy Guide.

- Nature of Healing
- Well-oiled bodies
- Lesser chemicals, better you

J. J. Lewis

Want more Bestseller Cook Books for **FREE?**

Join my **V.I.P** Reading List where I give away **Healthy** and Delicious Recipes **FOR FREE!**

Yes, you heard me right! COMPLETELY FREE to everyone just for being a loyal reader of mine!

http://www.ravenspress.com/jjlewis/

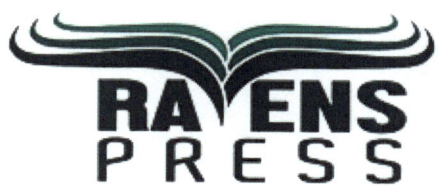

ISBN-13: 978-1515354055

ISBN-10: 1515354059

www.amazon.com/author/jjlewis

Table of Contents

introduction

There might be a lot of talk around you regarding essential oils and you are wondering what kinds of oils they might be. An essential oil is simply a liquid distilled from the flowers, leaves, roots, stems, bark and various elements of a plant. Most of the time, water or steam is used to distill these liquids. You may think that these essential oils have elements of oil in them due to the word "oil" but this is not the case.

Most of the essential oils are clear in color, although there are oils like orange, lemongrass and patchouli that can either have the yellow or amber color. Essential oils carry the true essence of the particular plants they are derived from. They are normally confused with perfume or fragrance oils yet they are quite different. Essential oils are created from true plants while perfume oils are derived from artificially created fragrances. The perfumes do not have the therapeutic benefits of essential oils.

There are various methods in which you can get the therapeutic benefits of essential oils. Examples include inhaling them or applying them directly on the skin. You can buy the various essential oils because they offer different benefits. The great thing about essential oils is that you can blend them together to be able to get all the different benefits at once. You can also purchase essential oils that have already been blended. The only disadvantage is that you have no control over the blending process and so you just have to do with the oils included.

What are essential oils?

Essential oils are volatile constituents of plants. These evaporating chemicals are the things which provide the plants its aroma, the spicy scent of basil, sweet tart smell of grapefruit, etc. The chemical composition of the essential oils differed from plant to plant and also depends on the region where it is grown.

Most of the essential oils are quite complex and are made up plenty of individual molecular components. Essential oils are extracted from the oil sacs in flowers, leaves, roots, stems, wood and bark. They differ from the regular vegetable oil, which is made of different fatty acids.

These essential oils help us in fighting infections, initiate cellular regeneration and work as a defense against fungus, virus, bacteria, etc. They have the same structure which is similar to the compounds found in your blood and tissues and hence they are compatible with our body physiology.

Essential oils of therapeutic quality are extracted very gently which will draw the oil from a particular plant. Extraction method can be:
· Carbon dioxide extraction- most gentle one and most expensive too
· Pressing
· Steam distillation
· Solvent extraction.

Steam distillation is a common way and requires only heating to a little above the boiling point of water, which is enough for most of the essential oils.

History

Humans have used plants for healing for thousands of years and from this the tradition of using aromatic plant compounds in medicine began. The use of aromatic plants was documented in 4500 B.C, though it was the Ancient Egyptians who developed oils and plant aromatics. Oils were used for purification rituals and in medicine. In 1922, when King Tut's tomb was opened in 1922, 50 alabaster jars were found that were to contain 350 liters of oil.

Over 200 references to aromatics, ointments and incense are mentioned in the Old and New Testaments. Some oils such as Cinnamon, Cassia, Frankincense, Myrrh, Spikenard and Rosemary were noted for being used for healing the sick and anointing rituals.

The first distillation of essential oil in the modern day was performed by the Persian philosopher Avicenna, who extracted the essence of the rose petals through effleurage process. In Mid 1500's, many aromatic botanicals were distilled in the Middle East and Europe. The term aromatherapy was coined in the middle of the last century by French chemist Rene-Maurice Gattefosse.

There are about 300 essential oils in use today by professionals, and on average a household can do with 10.

Benefits of essential oils

Essential oils contain numerous benefits and we are going to look at some of them.

1. Are able to penetrate your skin immediately

One of the benefits of essential oils is the fact that they are able to penetrate through your skin and cell membranes immediately. It only takes seconds for them to diffuse through your blood and tissues. These oils have the ability to get through the brain-blood barrier in order to get to the amygdala and various limbic parts of the brain. These are the parts that are in charge of controlling our mood, beliefs and emotions. This means that essential oils are capable of changing these three in order to enable us cope with stress, anger and the various emotions we are facing.

2. They have oxygenating properties

Essential oils contain oxygen molecules. They can therefore transport this oxygen to other cells in our bodies that are deprived of oxygen and to cells that need nutrients too. The cells in our body need oxygen to be healthy in order to be able to perform their functions properly and essential oils help with this.

3. They soothe muscles and joints

If you are suffering from aching muscles and joints, then essential oils might be a good remedy for that. You may have minor aches and pains due to the everyday activities you engage in and essential oils can still help to take care of this. When you combine them with a massage then you get even better results.

4. They contain high levels of antioxidants
Essential oils have been known to contain high level of antioxidants, which help the body.

Antioxidants are responsible for strengthening your body's system. This enables the body to prevent the negative effects that diet, aging and the environment have on our bodies. They also do away with free radicals. If you want to know the antioxidant capacity that essential oil contain then look at the ORAC (Oxygen Radical Absorbance Capacity) value indicated. For example, clove essential oil's ORAC value is 1, 078, 700 µTE/100g. This is very high compared to the one for carrots, which is at 210 µTE/100g.

5. They soothe digestion

Essential oils have been known to soothe digestion. Peppermints also known as Mentha Piperita are great herbs known for soothing digestions. They can also help to restore your digestive efficiency.

6. Are convenient and easy to use.

Essential oils are quite convenient in the sense that you can use them anywhere. Did you know that you could wear essential oils during the day? Yes, it is true and you can do this whether you are at home or work place. You can even carry them in your pocket.

These oils are important in massage too and they can improve your level of meditation and concentration.

7. Can be used on animals too

It's amazing that the use of essential oils is not limited to humans. Animals have been known to respond well to these oils too and great examples are dogs and horses. Although there are some limitations when it comes to cats, they can still be used on them.

8. Are safe for use

Essential oils have the ability to restore your body's balance without harming it. This is due to the fact that they do not contain any chemical based products. However, ensure to choose therapeutic grade essential oils and not the perfume grade ones because the latter is made of up harmful chemicals.

9. Multi –purpose

There are essential oils that perform more than one function. For example, true lavender essential oil also known, as Lavandula angustifolia is great for cuts and minor burns because it is gentle on the skin and contains antimicrobial properties too. It can also promote sleep and relaxation when inhaled. Therefore, you don't need to buy lots of essential oils.

10. Essential oils refine your skin

Using beauty products with lots of chemicals can sometimes diminish your natural glow. However, when you resort to essential oils then you can have it back. Essential oils help to give you a clear-looking complexion. In addition to that, they reduce the appearance of aging signs and give you healthy-looking hair.

11. Create a deep spiritual awareness

Essential oils have always been used in both spiritual and religious ceremonies. They help people to connect with a higher being than themselves. According to research, these essential oils have compounds that stimulate olfactory receptors. If you want to enhance your spiritual experience, then you can dilute the essential oils and apply them directly to your feet, wrists, behind the ears or let them diffuse in a quiet environment where you want to have your spiritual meditation.

How to choose and use essential oils

You may know about the benefits you stand to gain from essential oils but have no idea how to begin using them. Do not worry because this essential oils guide helps you figure out how to choose and then use essential oils.

What you have to know about essential oils before you buy them is that they serve different purposes and so you should make your choice based on what function you would like it to perform. For example, there are essential oils responsible for treating burns, elevating your mood and so on. It is important to find out more about the different essential oils and how you can identify the one you need. A good place to start is by reading. There are essential oils books available that can help you find the particular essential oil suitable for your particular need. While doing this, it is important to read about the cautions provided for each essential oil and the methods of application. We are going to look at some examples, although it is quite important to dilute the oils as instructed. Monitor your reaction to these oils and watch out for any adverse effects.

There are many questions that people normally ask about essential oils to give them a better understanding of what they entail and how to use them.

How should I use the essential oils?
There are three ways in which essential oils can get into your body. You can inhale them,

apply them on your skin or ingest them. These three ways are broken down into many kinds of methods used to apply them. For example, you can use spray, compresses, massage or baths to apply them on your skin.

How should I choose a method of application?

We've already established that there are many methods of application and you may wonder how to choose the most suitable one for you. There are factors you need to consider to help you make this choice and they are, the type of essential oil you want to use and the desired effect you hope to achieve. For example, wound care requires topical applications most of the time; baths need both topical absorption and inhalation while inhalation and topical application are recommended for mood effects. In case you are not sure of the application method you should use then it is advisable to consult an experienced aroma therapist.

How should I go about inhaling the essential oils?

There are various devices and techniques used to inhale essential oils.

Diffuser

Essential oils are normally placed inside the diffuser. Water may be added too, and even heat to help it evaporate. However, it is important to read the instructions first, don't just include the water and heat automatically. If you are advised to put it under heat, it is important to know that essential oils should not be subjected to direct heat because this will change their chemical structure. Diffusers are different and there are some with timers for convenience. Get instructions on how to use the one you have.

Dry evaporation

Put several drops of the essential oil on a piece of tissue or cotton ball and let it evaporate into the air. If your aim is to get an intense dose of the essential oils then you can try sniffing the cotton ball. If your aim is a milder dose, then you can have the cotton within your vicinity. For example, you can put it on your desk when you are on your computer.

Steam

Add some drops of the essential oil you are using in a bowl of steaming water. This will make the oil to vaporize. Cover your head and the bowl of water using a towel and breathe deeply.

Try not to use more than 2 drops of the essential oils because this method is quite direct and too much of it might be overwhelming. Make sure you keep your eyes closed during this method. This method is not recommended for children under 7 years old. Children above 7 years who need to use this method should cover their eyes with swimming goggles for protection purposes.

Spray.

Put drops of the essential oils in a water-based solution. Shake it and then spray in the air in order to set a good mood and deodorize the room. For example, if you want to portray the holiday feeling in a room, then you can use a solution of citrus oils to do this. Ensure you shake the bottle before you spray it to avoid a situation where you spray the water and not the solution, which might have settled at the bottom.

How are essential oils applied topically?

There are a variety of techniques that can be used to apply essential oils topically. What you should have at the back of your mind is that most of the essential oils, are not meant to be directly applied to your skin. That is why they are normally diluted first.

How are solutions prepared?

The rule of preparing solutions is that you should always dilute essential oils in a carrier substance. Examples of the carrier substances you can use include water or nut or vegetable oil. Their concentration shouldn't be more than 3-5%. When using the solution for massage or when you want to apply it over large sections of your body, then a 1% solution is recommended. This is about a drop of the essential oil in case you are using one teaspoon of carrier. 0.25% is enough for infants and 0.5% for toddlers. It is important to shake the solution in this case too before applying it.

Which carrier oils are suitable?

It is easy to get common carrier oils in stores that sell natural body and bath products. There are even natural food stores that have them. However, cold-pressed and organic oils are recommended and examples of these include apricot kernel, jojoba oil, almond oil, avocado oil and grape-seed oil. These oils have a mild smell of their own. These oils should be refrigerated until when you want to use them. In case you notice any rancid smell from them, then you should throw them away. They can stay for about a year when refrigerated before giving of the bad smell.

What are the techniques?

Compress.

The first step is diluting the essential oil in a liquid carrier (you can choose oil or water) before being applied directly to the affected place or to a dressing. You can apply heat or cold. An example includes adding some drops of ginger essential oil to hot water and mixing it. You can soak a piece of cloth in the mixture and put on your stiff joint. You can apply some heat if you wish.

Gargle.

Add drops of essential oil to the water and then mix it before gargling the solution. Make sure you do not swallow it, spit it out instead. You can do this if you are having a sore throat and tea tree oil is great for this purpose.

Bath.

Add drops of essential oils to your bath water, which is in a dispersant. Step into the bath water. Your skin will be able to absorb these oils and inhale the volatilized essential oil. Full cream milk can act as a dispersant and a few tablespoons are enough. When doing this, keep in mind that essential oils will float on the bath water because they are not water-soluble. You will able to capture the full strength of the essential oils when you pass through them. Bath salts can also disperse essential oils. You can use one part, two parts and three parts of baking soda, Epsom salts and sea salt respectively to come up with a relaxing bath base. Mix together this solution and true lavender essential oil in a ratio of 2 to 6 tablespoons and drops respectively. Mix it with your bath water and get in.

Massage.

Choose natural carrier oils and add drops of essential oil to it. Rub it gently on your skin. Stick to the same quantity mentioned in the introduction of "how solutions are prepared".

How are oils applied internally?

There is an internal application of essential oils and this can be done in various ways. Examples include suppositories and oral ingestion. However, you have to know that this method is only allowed in the U.S when supervised by a licensed healthcare provider.

How to use Essential oils as Herbal Medicine and Natural Remedies

Essential oils can be used in daily life in the form of herbal medicine and natural remedies and they are effective in treating many common ailments and preventing a lot more. Here is a guide on how you can use essential oils as herbal medicine and natural remedies:

Essential oils as a natural remedy

Aromatherapy has been used for thousands of years as medicines with a lot of healing properties. Essential oils can be used to improve physical and emotional health and restore balance to the whole body. It is an alternative medicine and they must be applied topically or inhaled.

When essential oils are diluted properly and used correctly you can enjoy the efficacy of aromatherapy. Essential oils can be used in the form of massage, steam inhalation, vaporizers, creams, lotions, mouthwashes, etc. It is essential that you determine the appropriate essential oil for your ailment. If you are not sure then you must contact a local aroma therapist. Here are top 10 essential oils which can be used for daily remedies:

1. Peppermint oil- This essential oil is known for its remedy for the digestive ailments such as indigestion, slow digestion, nausea, flatulence etc. It stimulates your liver, nervous system and your intestines. It can also reduce headaches, muscle aches and toothaches.

2. Eucalyptus- eucalyptus is a great essential oil, which is an effective decongestant for respiratory ailments such as colds, coughs, chest infections and sinusitis. It reduces fever, treats infections and reduces burn pains. It relieves muscle tension and fibrosis. It helps in forming new tissue and boosts your immunity.

3. Rosemary- It is a refreshing and stimulating oil. It has the capacity to improve your immunity, mental capacity, blood circulation and functions of the digestive system. It stimulates the nervous system and acts as an anti-depressant. It also has anti-bacterial, anti-fungal properties.

4. Lavender- This essential oil has calming, soothing and relaxing properties. It acts as an antiseptic, antibacterial and a painkiller which treats cuts, wounds, burns, allergies and insect bites. It has a balancing effect, reduces your blood pressure, and treats indigestion and nausea. Lavender essential oil also has the properties to treat depression, anxiety, stress and hypertension.

5. Lemon- This essential oil stimulates the body to fight infections, treat inflammation of the gums, mouth ulcers, acne, sore throat, etc. It helps fight against colds, flu and other respiratory ailments. It acts as a diuretic, laxative and astringent. Its pleasant and aromatic smell brightens your mood and calms your nerves. It fights anxiety and depression.

6. Ylang Ylang- It has sedative properties, is a good anti-depressant and a good tonic for the nervous system. It reduces anxiety, tensions and stress. It treats depressions and insomnia. It reduces blood pressure and slows your breathing and heart rate.

7. Tea tree- This essential oil has healing properties because it has anti-fungal, anti-viral and anti-bacterial properties. This oil is used to treat skin problems such as acne, warts, spots, blemishes, rashes, burn and blisters. It can clean wounds, infections, cuts and heal scar tissue. It can also boost the immunity and reduce inflammation. It also promotes relaxation and balances your hormones.

8. Geranium- this is in general called a feminine oil as it balances women's hormones. It can treat post-menopausal syndrome and other menopausal problems. This essential oil is refreshing and relaxing and it alleviates the symptoms of stress, anxiety and depression. It is a good anti-inflammatory and astringent which can balance the skin and relieve acne, burns, eczema, cuts and blocked pores.

9. Clary sage- This essential oil acts as an antidepressant and helps in treating depression, anxiety and other stress related issues. It can relieve muscle pains, pain and tension. It regulates the nervous system and also cures digestive system problems such as digestive spasms, flatulence and digestive spasms. It can also remove the excess oil on the skin. It can treat throat and respiratory infections.

10. Roman Chamomile- This essential oil has calming and relaxing properties and hence it can reduce anxiety, insomnia, tension and stress. It has anti-bacterial, anti-inflammatory and anti-septic properties. Chamomile can treat skin ailments such as allergies, boils, insect bites, rashes, wounds, infections etc. It can also relieve pain, toothaches, neuralgia, flatulence, indigestion, etc.

Essential oils as herbal medicine for some common problems

Therapeutic grade essential oils come in many varieties and blends and they have the ability to address many health conditions. Essential oils act as herbal medicine and you can treat many common problems with them. The following are some ailments to support our body systems:

Acne
· Tea Tree oil is a good choice for acne. It is equal to benzoyl peroxide which is used to treat acne.
· Gently massage a few drops of tea tree oil in the acne prone area twice a day.
· Other essential oils to treat acne are geranium, vetiver, Roman chamomile, cedar wood, rosewood, eucalyptus, orange, patchouli etc.

- Some good blends are Melorise and Purification.
- When the acne is infected, use clove essential oil
- Use lavender oil for scarring.

Allergies
- Essential oils are good for allergies; food, pollen and animal hair.
- Some essential oils for treating allergies are Lavender, Roman Chamomile, Eucalyptus, peppermint and lemon.
- These essential oils can boost your immune system.

Hay fever
- Hay fever is a general term which refers to allergic reactions caused due to airborne allergens such as feathers, chemicals, pollen or dust mites etc.
- These allergens trigger the release of histamines which can inflammation of the nasal passages which can cause sneezing, breathing difficulty, watery eyes etc.
- Lavender essential oil can be a good herbal medicine for treating hay fever and this can apply topically or aromatically.

Cat allergies
- Some kids are allergic to pets, especially cats and for this lavender essential oil is very effective.
- Other essential oil are peppermint, German chamomile and a blend like Raven and harmony.
- For rashes Roman chamomile, peppermint and elemi can be used.

Athlete's foot
- This is a fungal infection of the skin which affects the feet.
- Essential oils for athlete's foot are lavender, tea tree oil, thyme, blue cypress and mountain savory.
- Other essential oils blends for athlete's foot are Melrose, Thieves and Purification.

Bladder infection
- Add a drop of the essential oil blend Thieves to a glass of water and drink it many times a day.
- You can also massage the essential oil, juniper, lemongrass, tea tree, clove, oregano, thyme etc.
- Apply a warm compress after using these essential oils.

Cold sores
- Cold sores can be treated with lavender, peppermint, Melissa, frankincense, ravensara, rosewood, tea tree, sandalwood etc.
- Essential blends such as lemon and geranium, Melrose and purification can be used to

treat cold sores.

· Whether you are using a single essential oil or a blend, just apply one drop when you find the first sign of pain. Do this 5-10 times a day.

Chicken pox

· To treat chicken pox, mix 5-10 drops of German Chamomile and lavender each to an ounce of Calamine lotion and apply twice a day.

· Mix 10 drops of lavender and Roman chamomile and 4 ounces of Calamine lotion wherever needed two times a day.

· Other essential oils which are worth applying are eucalyptus, tea tree and bergamot oil.

Constipation

· Essential oils which can provide relief for constipation are ginger, peppermint, fennel, anise seed, and tarragon essential oils.

· Mix 3-5 drops of peppermint oil with ¼ teaspoon of raw organic extra virgin coconut oil in the bottom of a tea cup. Now add hot water and honey and drink it.

Joint pain

· Essential oils soothe joint pain and are applied topically by applying a few drops to the sore area.

· They can be applied diluted or undiluted to the sensitive skin. Some essential oils are spruce, German chamomile, pine, peppermint, wintergreen etc. Blends are Deep Relief, Pan Away and Aroma Siez.

Headaches

· Peppermint oil is the most common essential oil for treating headaches.

· Take a drop of this oil and rub it on your forehead, temples and back of your neck.

· Wintergreen oil also helps in natural headaches as it contains Salicylic acid, making it a pain reliever.

· You can also try the blend Aroma Life.

Sinus Congestion

· Put a couple of drops of peppermint oil on the scalp while inhaling deeply. Press peppermint oil drops on your tongue and press it to the roof of the mouth.

· Apply peppermint or eucalyptus oils to the reflex point on your feet.

· Other essential oils are tea tree, rosemary, thieves etc.

Sleep difficulties

· If you are troubled with insomnia, you can use lavender oil and blends such as Peace and Calming.

· These essential oils will decrease anxiety and promote tranquility.

Stress

· Many essential oils can be used to treat stress.

· Single oils which can be used for treating stress are lavender, Roman chamomile, cedar wood, sandalwood, valerian etc.

· Essential oil blends for relieving stress are peace and calming, valor, RutaVala, Tranquil and stress away.

The best way to apply these oils is topically or aromatically. To apply it topically take a few drops and rub it on your feet, chest, wrists etc. For aromatic purpose inhale it by opening the bottle and inhaling deeply or add it to a diffuser.

Essential Oil recipes for relaxation and stress relief

Stress has been proven to be one of the leading causes of many health problems and even deaths in extreme cases. The life we live today exposes us to higher risks of stress and this is why there has been an increase in the number of people looking for stress remedies. There are various methods used by different people to deal with stress and using essential oils is one of them.

Essential oils are known to give you a relaxing and calming effect, which we need in our busy lives. The essential oils do this with the use of aromatherapy.

There are some home remedies that you may use to create that happy and calming effect. You may wonder how aromatherapy is connected to stress reduction. Well, it stimulates limbic and endocrine systems and these are the systems responsible for your hormones and emotions. When this happens, it triggers both an emotional and physical response, which is positive in this case. An example is what happens if you happen to smell Lavender essential oil. The microscopic chemicals in it trigger your system, which responds by calming down your nervous system leading to relaxing of muscles.

There have been several studies conducted on the link between aromatherapy and stress reduction and the results were positive. It was discovered that people suffering from Alzheimer's disease were treated with lemon and lavender essential oils and this reduced their level of agitation. Depressed men took less anti-depressant after using citrus essential oils. Ylang Ylang essential oils were discovered to boost the production of endorphins in the body and these are the hormones responsible for reducing pain and giving you the feeling of being well. All these prove that aromatherapy works for stress reduction and relaxation.

Examples of the best essential oils to help you reduce stress and tension include lavender, marjoram, benzoin, geranium, Melissa, vanilla, orange, cinnamon, neroli, rose, Ylang Ylang and chamomile among others.

Strategies for aromatherapy stress relief

I know that you've told over and over again to take good care of yourself but I have to say it again. Self-care is essential in helping your body fight stress. Most of us say that we would like to take better care of ourselves but we don't have the time. However, when you really think about it, it will cost you more in terms of time and money if you don't take care of yourself. Just stop doing too much. If you start to feel out of control, then you can take small breaks during the day to calm yourself down. Doing this twice a day for about 5 minutes is enough. You can increase this amount of time later on to about 15 minutes when your tolerance level increases. If you find this difficult then you can try using the aromatherapy inhaler recipe.

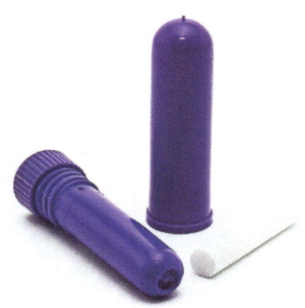

1. Making your own aromatherapy inhaler

Having your own aromatherapy inhaler is great because it is quite portable. You can therefore have it with you all the time because it is small and can fit in your bag, car and therefore can use it whenever the need arises.

Ingredients:
1 teaspoon of coarse sea salt.
10 Drops of Bergamot essential oil.
4 Drops of Orange essential oil.
4 Drops of Lavender essential oil.
1 Drop of Chamomile or Ylang Ylang essential oil.

1 Drop of Rose Geranium essential oil.
Glass bottles.

Procedure:
1. Pour the coarse sea salt in an extremely small and dark plastic bottle or glass.

2. Add all the other ingredients to it.

3. Inhale the aroma in three slow, deep breaths.

4. Relax for a while and inhale the aroma again in three deep breaths. Ensure you do this thrice and you will have great aromatherapy stress relief.

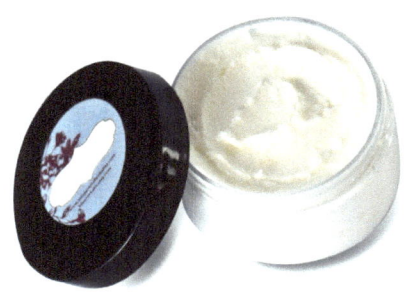

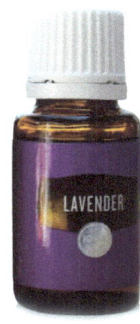

2. Scented mineral bath of Ylang Ylang and lemon

These essential oils are great for your senses. They are great because they are moderately relaxing and energizing and have a clean sweet fragrance.

Ingredients:
1 tablespoon of baking soda.
2 tablespoons of sea salt.
1-½ teaspoons of borax.
6 Drops of lemon essential oils.
4 Drops of Ylang Ylang.

Procedure:
1. Mix together the baking soda, sea salt, and borax.

2. Add the lemon and Ylang Ylang essential oils to the mixture and mix well.

3. Prepare a bath and pour the mixture inside under running water. Ensure the salts completely dissolve and the oils evenly dispersed in the water. You can add some drops of Lavender to create a good balance.

3. Lavender, Chamomile and Tangerine blend

This blend is great for relaxation and stress reduction. It will make your muscles, tissues and joints relax and give you a good energy balance.

Ingredients:
3 Drops of Tangerine.
3 Drops of Lavender.
3 Drops of Chamomile.
1 ounce of carrier oil. (Choose any)

Procedure:
1. Blend the above essential oils together in the carrier oil.

2. Massage as desired.
This blend can also act as bath oil.

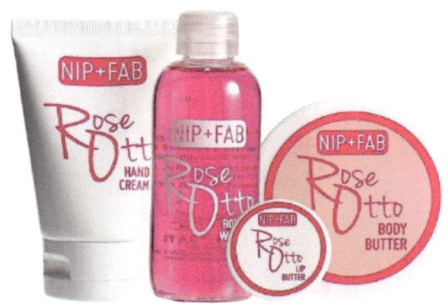

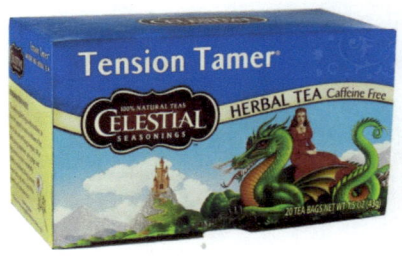

4. Rose Otto

This aroma is quite an effective aphrodisiac. It has benefits on both your mind and body. It has the ability to relax your spirit and relieve you of stress. You can enjoy it as a relaxing bath.

Ingredients:
Bath water.
3 ½ tablespoons of heavy cream.
3 Drops of the Turkish Rose-Otto essential oil.

Procedure:
1. Mix the heavy cream and Turkish Rose-Otto essential oil.

2. Add the mixture to the bath water.

5. Tension taming recipes

This aromatherapy bath salt recipe will help to ease away your tension. They do this by balancing your nervous system which affects your mood swings too. This recipe is quite good, especially for those with oily skin because it helps to cleanse the skin and reduce the production of oil in addition to healing blemished skin.

Ingredients
1 cup of sea salt.
3 Drops of the Lavender essential oil.
6 Drops of Bergamot essential oil.
½ cup of baking soda.
6 Drops of the sweet Orange essential oil.
4 Drops of yellow and 6 drops of red food coloring. (This is optional)

Procedure
1. Use a metal spoon to mix together the salt and baking soda. (A metal spoon is recommended because a wooden spoon will be ruined from absorbing the essential oils).

2. Pour drops of the essential oils on top of the salts and stir it until it is properly mixed. Do the same with the food coloring.

3. Keep the mixture in a plastic jar or dark glass and leave it for 24 hours before using it.

4. A cup of salt is enough for a single bath. This recipe you just made can last for three baths.
It is important to note that sweet orange and Bergamot should not be used before being exposed to the sun. This is due to the fact that they have the ability to cause sunburn and photosensitivity.

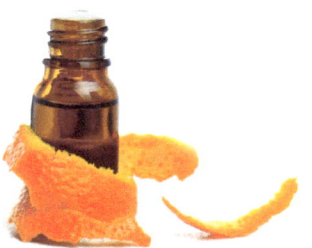

6. Aromatherapy bath oil recipe for relaxing

This recipe for bath oil is super relaxing and it will make you very calm and at peace. All you need to do is take some slow, deep breaths of it and all your stress will melt away. The deep scent of this bath oil is especially great for men. You can use it as massage oil for your man and this will help him relax to an extent that he might even fall asleep. Sandalwood essential oil is part of the ingredients used in this bath oil and it is important for healing the skin. Therefore, if you have skin conditions such as psoriasis and eczema then this bath oil is good for you. In addition to that, it helps to slow down the aging process and revitalizes your skin.

Ingredients
12 Drops of the Lavender essential oil.
4fl oz. equivalent of 125 ml of the carrier oil you prefer. Examples include almond and jojoba oil.
30 Drops of the Sandalwood essential oil.
2 Drops of Cedar wood essential oil.

Procedure
1. Mix all the ingredients together in a plastic bottle or dark glass. Store the bottle in a cool, dark place. (Keep it away from your bathroom because of the warmth and humidity)

2. Pour a tablespoon of the aromatherapy bath oil you made in the bath running after running it. It is as simple as that and you are ready to take that super-relaxing bath that will relieve your stress.

Be careful to avoid going for cheap Sandalwood because it will not give you the same results as the original one. It may be a bit expensive but it is worth your money.

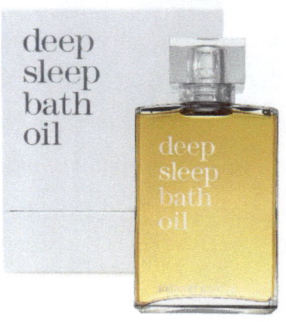

7. Aromatherapy bath oil for sweet dreams

This bath recipe is quite soothing and is especially good for people suffering from insomnia. This is because it will soothe you to sleep. If you are having one of those days where sleep is elusive then there is no need to worry. You can try out this bath oil, which will calm your nerves and relax your muscles. You will then be able to have a peaceful sleep when your mind is calm too. In addition to that, the essential oils will help to repair your skin and reduce the appearance of wrinkles. In case you are not able to take a bath, then you can massage your face and torso using some of the lavender oil and you will still enjoy its luxurious effect. It is advisable to do this before you get into bed in order to have a deep sleep.

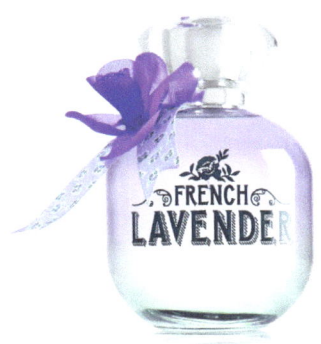

8. Lavender

Did you know that you could make your own massage oil? Well, it is possible. Although bath oils are important, you may not always have the time to take a bath. However, if you have the massage oil, then you can use it to get the same results. Lavender is pleasing to the eye, has an amazing scent and contains numerous healing powers so preparing Lavender massage oils is a good decision.

This massage oil is great for insomnia, pain, stress and anxiety. When you combine these amazing effects of Lavender with its gentle touch, you are on the right path to achieving an intense kind of relaxation. If you are not in a position to have a full body massage then you can even do some foot massage. This massage oil can also be rubbed on your chest and stomach to help you sleep.

Ingredients
2 Drop of the Clary Sage essential oil.
12 Drops of the Lavender essential oil.
3 Drops of Marjoram essential oil.
12 Drops of either Orange or Bergamot essential oil.
1 drop of Vetiver essential oil
¼ cup of any carrier oil you prefer.

Procedure
1. Mix all the ingredients together in a plastic bottle or dark glass. It is advisable to get a bottle or glass with a lotion or oil dispenser cup. This is to avoid accidental spillage.

2. Wait for a period of 24 hours before using the massage in order to give time to "cure". The bottle should be stored in a cool, dark place and used within three months.

You can either double or triple the quantity of the ingredients if you want to have a large amount of the massage oil.

One thing you have to remember when choosing carrier oils is that you can tailor them to suit your specific skin needs. It is advisable to choose the ones that help to nourish and support your skin. For example, if you are using jojoba or sweet almond oil, then you can add sea buckthorn oil or borage oil to it if you have dry or maturing skin. It is okay to experiment with the different carrier oils in order to find out what suits your skin best. This can be a fun experience.

Essential oils recipes for mental health

Our mental health is equally as important as our physical health if not more. This is due to the fact that our brain is always working every waking minute and yet it is what holds us together. If we overwork it or subject it to too much stress, then we are bound to lose our minds and no one would like that. There are essential oils that are known to improve your mental health. If you want to have a smarter, quicker and clearer brain, then essential oils are the way to go. If you open your mind to it, you will be amazed because you can experience the results immediately. These are the five essential oils known to improve your mental clarity.

· Rosemary
· Juniper Berry
· Sage or Clary Sage
· Basil
· Peppermint

There are several ways of using the essential oils to help clear your mind. One of the easiest ways of doing this is by dropping the essential oils inside a pot with lots of water. You can then heat the water until it is steaming before turning down the heat. You can just leave the pot on the burner and the essential oils will evaporate into the air, giving your home the sweet scents of the oil. If you find trouble sleeping at night and you don't want to wake up the whole family by filling the house with essential oils then you can use a candle diffuser. It is as easy as putting the essential oils in the top bowl before lighting a tea light below it.

The tea light will give off heat, which will make the essential oils evaporate into the air, and you will capture those amazing scents, which will soothe you to sleep.

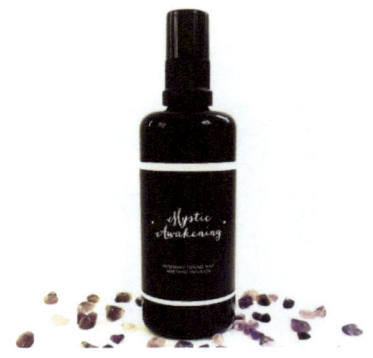

9. Rosemary Mist

This will serve to stimulate your senses and is great for after you have showered but just before you towel off. You need to use it when your skin is still damp.

Ingredients:
6 drops of the rosemary essential oil
Spray bottle.
1 teaspoon of olive oil.
5 ounces of distilled water.
1 sprig fresh rosemary

Procedure:
1. Add all the ingredients in the spray bottle and shake well in order for them to mix properly.

2. Spritz it on as you wish.

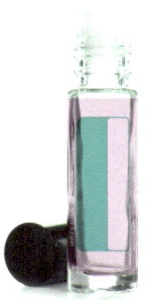 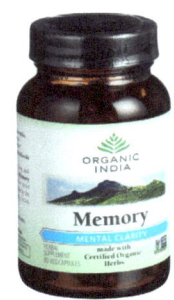

10. Alertness massage oil

This massage oil will help to improve your mental health by increasing your brain alertness.

Ingredients:
6 Drops of ginger.
4 Drops of Juniper Berry
5 Drops of Grapefruit.
 15 ml of your preferred carrier oil.

Procedure:
1. Mix all the ingredients together.

2. Take drops of it and use it to massage the back of your neck and your temples because it is ready for use.

11. Mental clarity spray

Mental clarity is part of great mental health and this is the purpose that the spray aims to achieve.

Ingredients:
50 Drops of lemongrass.
20 Drops of Cedar wood
40 Drops of Niaouli.
40 Drops of rosemary.
4 ounces, which is equivalent of 120 ml of pure water.

Procedure:
1. Mix together all the essential oils and then add water.

2. Shake well.

3. Put inside the sprayer ready for use whenever you need it.

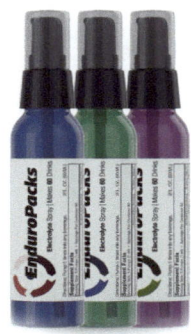

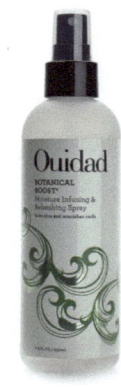

12. Alertness spray

When you use this spray, you will be more alert to be able to concentrate on what you are doing.

Ingredients:
40 Drops of Bergamot
25 Drops of Lavender
40 Drops of Grapefruit
30 Drops of Juniper Berry
40 Drops of Peppermint
4 ounces of pure water

Procedure:
1. Mix all the ingredients together inside a mist sprayer

2. Shake well.

3. Spray it from the mist sprayer.

13. Refreshing spray

Both our bodies and minds need to be refreshed every now and then to be able to take on more responsibilities.

Ingredients:
4 oz. of distilled water
10 Drops of Orange essential oil
5 ml of Emulsified essential oil
50 Drops of lime essential oil
50 Drops of Grapefruit essential oil

Procedure:
1. Mix together the emulsifier and all the essential oils in a clean bottle.
2. Add distilled water inside the bottle.
3. Shake the bottle well.
4. Spritz the contents in the air.

Remember to always shake the bottle before you spritz the contents. You can use these ingredients in any diffuser as long as you do away with the water and the emulsifier. You can use an amber bottle to blend it, then shake properly before placing some drops in your diffuser.
Blending the various essential oils yourself to serve different purposes is great because you have control over the ingredients you use. However, do not beat yourself up if you don't have the time to make them yourself. You can always buy them. Just ask for the particular essential

oils or the blends of essential blends that you need. Either way, you can benefit from them.

Acne & Blemished Skin

Acne is a skin condition that is caused by the over production of oil in the sebaceous glands. This excess oil mixes with dead cells on the surface of the skin, causing the follicle to become blocked. Bacteria, that are already present on the skin, contaminate the follicle resulting in the appearance of blackheads, pimples, whiteheads, nodules or cysts.

The most common treatments for acne are often prescribed antibiotics, harsh antibacterial face washes, and/or steroids. Over time, these can have a harmful effect on the skin, causing sensitization, facial swelling, redness, and irritation. As a result, many people turn to essential oils as an alternative holistic treatment, due to the powerful antibacterial and anti-inflammatory properties they possess.

Essential oils for acne & blemished skin; Benzoin, Bergamot, Cedar wood, Chamomile (German or Roman), Clary Sage, Geranium, Grapefruit, Juniper Berry, Lavender, Lemon, Lemongrass, Mandarin, Orange (Sweet), Rosemary, Tea Tree, Thyme.

Carrier oils for acne & blemished skin; Sweet Almond, Borage Seed, Coconut, Hazelnut.

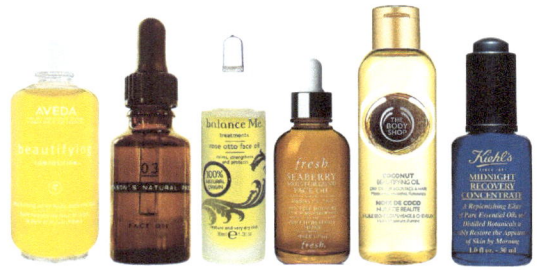

14. Facial Oils

Blend all the ingredients together and mix thoroughly. Apply the formula to a cleansed face and neck, and gently massage using small circular movements. Leave the oils to absorb into the skin cells, do not wash off. Carry out the treatment twice per day, once in the morning and again at night. At night, a facial oil can be substituted with a facial moisturizer (recipes below) if you prefer. The following recipes will yield enough for 1 treatment. Where coconut oil is used in these recipes, make sure to use Raw Virgin Coconut Oil as it is the best form of coconut oil to use for the skin. Melt it by placing an even tablespoon into a cup, place the cup in a saucepan of boiling water, and continue to boil the water on the heat until the coconut oil has melted. Never melt in the microwave.

Day Blend 1

1 tablespoon coconut oil
5 drops of tea tree
4 drops of lavender
1 drop of geranium

Day Blend 2

1 tablespoon jojoba oil
10 drops of tea tree

Day Blend 3

1 tablespoon borage seed oil

4 drops of chamomile

4 drops of thyme

2 drops of lavender

Day Blend 4

1 tablespoon coconut oil

4 drops of lemon

4 drops of geranium

2 drops of neroli

Night Blend 1

1 tablespoon sweet almond oil

6 drops of bergamot

6 drops of tea tree

3 drops of lemon

Night Blend 2

1 tablespoon borage seed oil

10 drops of tea tree

5 drops of lavender

Night Blend 3

1 tablespoon coconut oil

10 drops of rosemary

2 drops of grapefruit

2 drops of juniper

1 drop of lavender

Night Blend 4

1 tablespoon jojoba oil

8 drops of lemongrass

4 drops of chamomile

3 drops of tea tree

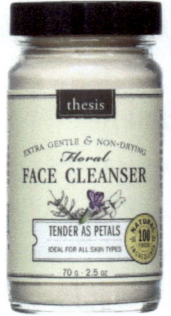

15. Facial Cleansers

Blend all ingredients together and mix thoroughly. Apply the formula to the face and neck, and massage into the skin using outward circular movements. Leave to absorb into the skin for 2 minutes. Gently remove all traces of oil, preferably using a wet muslin cloth soaked in warm water. A small, soft face towel can be used as an alternative. Repeat twice per day, once in the morning and again at night before applying a facial oil or moisturizer. The following recipes will yield enough for 1 treatment. Regarding coconut oil, please refer to 'Facial Oils' above for instructions on how to prepare. Where shea butter is used, melt it by placing an even tablespoon into a cup, place the cup in a saucepan of boiling water, and continue to boil the water on the heat until the shea butter has melted. Never melt in the microwave.

Blend 1

1 tablespoon aloe Vera gel

1 tablespoon coconut milk

8 drops of tea tree

4 drops of peppermint

2 drops of lavender

Blend 2

2 tablespoons raw honey

5 drops of rosemary

5 drops of lavender

5 drops of grapefruit

Blend 3

2 tablespoons extra virgin olive oil

4 drops of lemon

4 drops of grapefruit

2 drops of peppermint

2 drops of tea tree

Blend 4

1 tablespoon coconut milk

1 teaspoon coconut oil

15 drops of tea tree

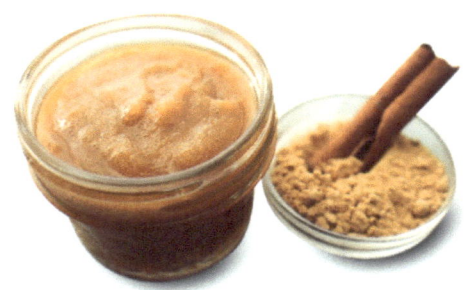

16. Facial Scrubs

Combine all ingredients in a small bowl, mix thoroughly and use immediately. Massage the blend gently into the skin as you would the facial cleanser. Leave on the skin for 2 minutes and wash off with warm water. Carry out this treatment once per week. The following recipes will yield enough for 1 treatment. Regarding coconut oil, please refer to 'Facial Oils' above for instructions on how to prepare.

Blend 1

1 tablespoon baking soda

1 teaspoon water

10 drops of tea tree

2 drops of lavender

2 drops of chamomile

Blend 2

1 teaspoon brown sugar

6 drops of rosemary

5 drops of bergamot

2 drops of grapefruit

2 drops of geranium

Blend 3

½ cup ground oatmeal

1 tablespoon raw honey

1 teaspoon jojoba oil

6 drops of benzoin

6 drops of tea tree

6 drops of rosemary

Blend 4
1 teaspoon baking soda
1 teaspoon fresh lemon juice
1 teaspoon olive oil
4 drops of frankincense
4 drops of sandalwood
2 drops of lavender
2 drops of tea tree
2 drops of chamomile

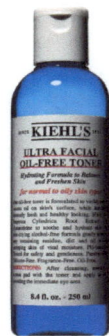

17. Facial Toners

Blend all ingredients in a glass bottle and shake well to combine. You can use a spray bottle if you wish but it is not necessary. Always add the hydrosol (flower water) first and then follow with the essential oils. Distilled water is a great alternative to hydrosols but always ensure you use distilled water (tap water may contain chemicals or bacteria). If you are using a spray bottle, hold it 3 to 4 inches away from the face, close your eyes and spray. Do not wipe off. If you are using a normal bottle, soak a cotton pad with the toner and gently pat all over the face and neck. Apply each time after cleansing, exfoliating or a face mask. The following recipes will yield enough for approximately 2 to 3 days.

Blend 1
½ cup cold green tea
½ cup apple cider vinegar
10 drops of tea tree

Blend 2
1 cup distilled water
10 drops of rosemary
5 drops of bergamot

Blend 3
1 cup witch hazel
4 drops of geranium
4 drops of lemongrass

4 drops of tea tree

Blend 4
½ cup distilled water
Juice from 1 lemon
4 drops of grapefruit
4 drops of tea tree
4 drops of orange (sweet)
2 drops of peppermint

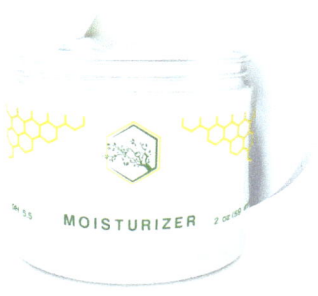

18. Facial Moisturizers

Blend all ingredients together and mix thoroughly. After cleansing and toning, apply the formula onto the face and neck, and massage into the skin, using small, gentle circular movements with the fingertips. If you are applying a day blend, allow the oils to absorb into the skin for 2 minutes before applying makeup. Repeat twice per day, once in the morning and again at night. A moisturizer may be substituted for a facial oil (recipes above) if you wish. The following recipes will yield enough for 1 - 2 treatments. Regarding coconut oil, please refer to 'Facial Oils' above for instructions on how to prepare.

Blend 1
5 tablespoons jojoba oil
7 tablespoons coconut oil
2 tablespoons aloe Vera gel
* mix the above ingredients in a blender. Once blended, scoop out, and add;
15 drops of tea tree
5 drops of lavender
2 drops of chamomile
2 drops of bergamot
2 drops of rosemary

Blend 2
2 tablespoons shea butter
1 tablespoon rosehip seed oil
2 vitamin E capsules

*mix the above ingredients in a blender. Once blended, scoop out, and add;
8 drops of frankincense
8 drops of grapefruit
6 drops of sandalwood
2 drops of lavender

Blend 3
2 tablespoons aloe Vera gel
4 tablespoons jojoba oil
Juice from ½ lemon
1 tablespoon coconut milk
*mix the above ingredients in a blender. Once blended, scoop out, and add;
20 drops of tea tree

Blend 4
½ cup distilled water
1 teaspoon fresh lemon juice
1 tablespoon extra-virgin olive oil
1 tablespoon jojoba oil
*mix the above ingredients in a blender. Once blended, scoop out, and add;
6 drops of lemon
6 drops of lavender
4 drops of grapefruit
2 drops of bergamot

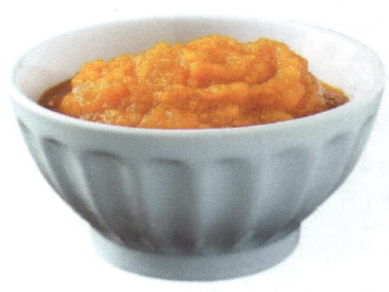

19. v

Blend all ingredients in a small bowl, mix thoroughly and use immediately. Apply the formula with either a mask brush or clean fingers, after the skin has been cleansed. Leave on for 15 to 20 minutes and wash off with warm water. Pat dry the face, follow with a toner and moisturizer or facial oil. Apply a face mask once every week. The following recipes will yield enough for 1 treatment.

Blend 1
2 tablespoons raw honey
1 tablespoon apple cider vinegar
4 drops of frankincense
4 drops of chamomile
4 drops of thyme
4 drops of tea tree

Blend 2
1 small ripe banana (mashed)
1 tablespoon raw honey
2 teaspoons fresh lemon juice
10 drops of tea tree
6 drops of chamomile
4 drops of clary sage

Blend 3
2 egg whites
Juice from ½ lemon
6 drops of benzoin

6 drops of bergamot

2 drops of cypress

2 drops of chamomile

Blend 4

4 tablespoons coconut oil

1 tablespoon raw honey

1 tablespoon baking soda

10 drops of chamomile

5 drops of lavender

Blend 5

2 tablespoons raw honey

1 teaspoon cinnamon

Juice from ¼ lemon

5 drops of thyme

5 drops of benzoin

5 drops of tea tree

Blend 6

2 tablespoons plain yogurt

1 tablespoon aloe Vera gel

1 teaspoon jojoba oil

5 drops of tea tree

2 drops of bergamot

2 drops of grapefruit

2 drops of lavender

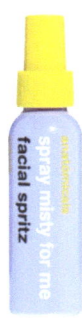

20. Facial Spritz

Blend all ingredients together in a spray bottle and mix thoroughly. Hold the bottle 3-4 inches from the face, close your eyes and spritz liberally. Repeat several times per day.

Blend 1

50ml distilled water

15 drops of tea tree

Blend 2

50ml lavender hydrosol

5 drops of chamomile

5 drops of benzoin

5 drops of lavender

Blend 3

50ml distilled water

2 tablespoons aloe Vera juice

10 drops of bergamot

5 drops of rosemary

Blend 4

40ml distilled water

1 tablespoon apple cider vinegar

1 tablespoon fresh lemon juice

2 drops of geranium

2 drops of clary sage

2 drops of chamomile

2 drops of juniper berry

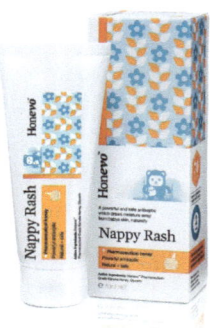

21. Topical Treatments

Tea tree and lavender are the only 2 essential oils recommended for direct use on blemishes. It is always advised to apply with a cotton bud as bacteria may be present on the fingertips. If you do not have cotton buds to hand, make sure and wash your hands thoroughly before application. Once applied, there is no need to wash off. Essential oils can cause irritation to the skin if overused, particularly tea tree in undiluted form, therefore topical treatments should only be carried out 2-4 times per week.

Blend 1
Apply 2 drops of tea tree on a cotton bud and gently tap the pimple.

Blend 2
Apply 1 drop of lavender and 1 drop of tea tree on a cotton bud and gently tap the pimple.

Age Spots

Age spots, also known as brown spots or liver spots, are flat, brown areas of pigmentation that vary in size and usually appear on the face, hand, neck, arms and shoulders. They are caused by excessive exposure to the sun, and while they are very common in maturing adults, they can affect younger people as well. Over time, essential oils can lighten age spots and in some cases completely remove them.

Essential oils for age spots; Cypress, Frankincense, Geranium, Grapefruit, Lavender, Lemon, Myrrh, Sandalwood, Ylang Ylang.

Carrier oils for age spots; Coconut (raw virgin), Evening Primrose, Jojoba.

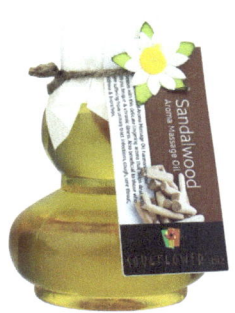

22. Massage Oils

Blend all ingredients together and mix thoroughly. Apply to the age spot, or if there is a cluster of them, apply to the whole area. Leave to absorb into the skin, do not wash off. Repeat daily. When using coconut oil, it is recommended to use Raw Virgin Coconut Oil. The following recipes provide treatments for 1 week.

Blend 1

1 tablespoon raw virgin coconut oil
5 drops of myrrh
5 drops of frankincense
5 drops of lavender
*melt the coconut oil first, add essential oils and leave to solidify.

Blend 2

2 tablespoons jojoba oil
10 drops of frankincense
5 drops of sandalwood

Blend 3

1 tablespoon aloe Vera gel
10 drops of sandalwood
2 drops of lemon
2 drops of cypress
1 drop of lavender

Blend 4

1 tablespoon coconut oil
8 drops of frankincense
4 drops of geranium
2 drops of grapefruit
1 drop of Ylang Ylang

Aging/Mature Skin

Believe it or not the skin of individuals aged over 25 years is termed mature skin. Once we hit our mid-twenties, collagen and elastin (proteins that keep the skin firm and supple) production in our skin cells starts to slow down. As a result the skin starts to develop signs of aging, including loss of elasticity, the appearance of fine lines and wrinkles, reduced muscle tone, thinner skin, and age spots, dilated capillaries and skin tags become more apparent. While these changes in the skin are a natural part of aging, essential oils help to slow down the aging process, keeping the skin looking younger and healthier for longer.

Essential oils for aging/mature skin; Frankincense, Geranium, Jasmine, Lavender, Myrrh, Neroli, Patchouli, Sandalwood, Rose, Rosewood.

Carrier oils for aging/mature skin; Sweet Almond, Avocado, Coconut (raw virgin), Evening Primrose, Jojoba, Rosehip Seed (not really a carrier oil as such but a fantastic nourishing and regenerating oil for the skin).

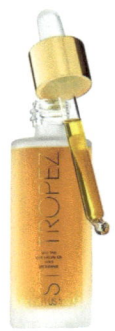

23. Facial Oils

Blend all the ingredients together and mix thoroughly. Apply the formula to a cleansed face and neck, and gently massage using small circular movements. Leave the oils to absorb into the skin cells, do not wash off. Carry out the treatment twice per day, once in the morning and again at night. At night, a facial oil can be substituted with a facial moisturizer (recipes below) if you prefer. The following recipes will yield enough for 1 treatment. Wherqae coconut oil is used in these recipes, make sure to use Raw Virgin Coconut Oil as it is the best form of coconut oil to use for the skin. Melt it by placing an even tablespoon into a cup, place the cup in a saucepan of boiling water, and continue to boil the water on the heat until the coconut oil has melted. Never melt in the microwave.

Blend 1

2 tablespoons melted coconut oil

6 drops of frankincense

5 drops of geranium

2 drops of neroli

2 drops of rose

Blend 2

2 tablespoons jojoba oil

6 drops of myrrh

6 drops of sandalwood

3 drops of jasmine

Blend 3

1 tablespoon avocado oil

1 teaspoon rosehip seed oil

5 drops of frankincense

5 drops of myrrh

3 drops of sandalwood

2 drops of lavender

Blend 4

1 tablespoon coconut oil

1 teaspoon rosehip seed oil

6 drops of neroli

4 drops of rose

4 drops of frankincense

1 drop of jasmine

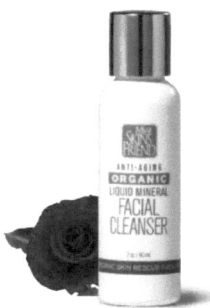

24. Facial Cleansers

Blend all ingredients together and mix thoroughly. Apply the formula to the face and neck, and massage into the skin using outward circular movements. Leave to absorb into the skin for 2 minutes. Gently remove all traces of oil, preferably using a wet muslin cloth soaked in warm water. A small, soft face towel can be used as an alternative. Repeat twice per day, once in the morning and again at night before applying a facial oil or moisturizer. The following recipes will yield enough for 1 treatment. Regarding coconut oil, please refer to 'Facial Oils' above for instructions on how to prepare. Where shea butter is used, melt it by placing an even tablespoon into a cup, place the cup into a saucepan of boiling water, and continue to boil the water on the heat until the shea butter has melted. Never melt in the microwave.

Blend 1
1 tablespoon jojoba oil
1 teaspoon melted coconut oil (raw virgin)
6 drops of carrot seed
6 drops of frankincense
3 drops of sandalwood

Blend 2
1 tablespoon aloe Vera gel
1 vitamin E capsule
5 drops of jasmine
5 drops of rosemary
5 drops of lavender

Blend 3
1 tablespoon evening primrose
1 tablespoon melted coconut oil
8 drops of lavender
2 drops of geranium
2 drops of carrot seed
2 drops of myrrh
1 drop of rose

Blend 4
1 tablespoon cocoa butter
1 teaspoon rosehip seed oil
6 drops of clary sage
4 drops of lemon
4 drops of geranium
1 drop of neroli

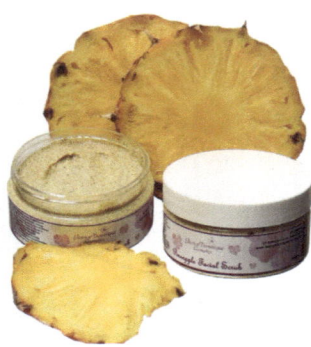

25. Facial Scrubs

Combine all ingredients in a small bowl, mix thoroughly and use immediately. Massage the blend gently into the skin as you would the facial cleanser. Leave on the skin for 2 minutes and wash off with warm water. Carry out this treatment once per week. The following recipes will yield enough for 1 treatment. Regarding coconut oil, please refer to 'Facial Oils' above for instructions on how to prepare.

Blend 1

1 tablespoon plain natural yogurt

1 teaspoon ground oatmeal

1 teaspoon melted coconut oil

5 drops of jasmine

2 drops of myrrh

1 drop of patchouli

Blend 2

1 tablespoon ground oatmeal

1 tablespoon coconut milk

1 vitamin E capsule

4 drops of chamomile

4 drops of frankincense

Blend 3

1 tablespoon mashed papaya

1 teaspoon manuka honey

6 drops of frankincense

2 drops of lavender

Blend 4

1 tablespoon manuka honey

1 teaspoon ground almonds

4 drops of rosemary

3 drops of geranium

1 drop of neroli

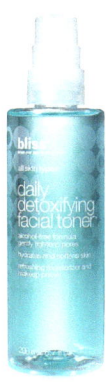

Blend 3

50ml distilled water

10 drops of frankincense

10 drops of geranium

Blend 4

50ml rose water

15 drops of rose

10 drops of neroli

26. Facial Toners

Blend all ingredients in a glass bottle and shake well to combine. You can use a spray bottle if you wish but it is not necessary. Always add the hydrosol (flower water) first and then follow with the essential oils. Distilled water is a great alternative to hydrosols but always ensure you use distilled water (tap water may contain chemicals or bacteria). If you are using a spray bottle, hold it 3 to 4 inches away from the face, close your eyes and spray. Do not wipe off. If you are using a normal bottle, soak a cotton pad with the toner and gently pat all over the face and neck. Apply each time after cleansing, exfoliating or a face mask. The following recipes will yield enough for approximately 2 to 3 days.

Blend 1

50ml distilled water

10 drops of lavender

5 drops of rosewood

5 drops of jasmine

5 drops of patchouli

Blend 2

50ml rose water

20ml aloe Vera juice

10 drops of frankincense

10 drops of rose

5 drops of geranium

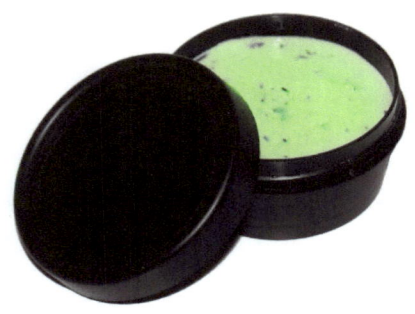

27. Facial Masks

Blend all ingredients in a small bowl, mix thoroughly and use immediately. Apply the formula with either a mask brush or clean fingers, after the skin has been cleansed. Leave on for 15 to 20 minutes and wash off with warm water. Pat dry the face, follow with a toner and moisturizer or facial oil. Apply a face mask once every week. The following recipes will yield enough for 1 treatment.

Blend 1
½ ripe avocado, mashed
1 teaspoon rosehip seed oil
5 drops of frankincense
5 drops of rosemary
5 drops of myrrh

Blend 2
1 tablespoon manuka honey
1 tablespoon evening primrose
8 drops of carrot seed
4 drops of sandalwood
3 drops of rose

Blend 3
1 tablespoon cocoa powder
1 vitamin E capsule
1 teaspoon coconut milk
1 teaspoon rosehip seed oil
Mix into a paste and then add;

6 drops of clary sage
4 drops of rosemary
3 drops of geranium
2 drops of lavender

Blend 4
1 tablespoon aloe Vera gel
1 teaspoon avocado oil
1 teaspoon jojoba oil
6 drops of jasmine
6 drops of cedar wood
2 drops of neroli
1 drop of lavender

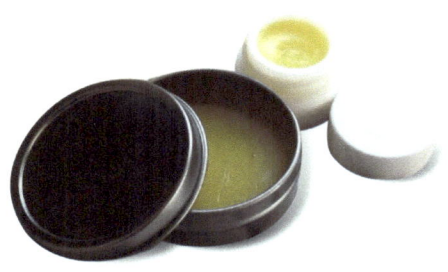

28. Facial Moisturizers

Blend all ingredients together and mix thoroughly. After cleansing and toning, apply the formula onto the face and neck, and massage into the skin, using small, gentle circular movements with the fingertips. If you are applying a day blend, allow the oils to absorb into the skin for 2 minutes before applying makeup. Repeat twice per day, once in the morning and again at night. A moisturizer may be substituted for a facial oil (recipes above) if you wish. The following recipes will yield enough for 1 - 2 treatments. Regarding coconut oil, please refer to 'Facial Oils' above for instructions on how to prepare.

Blend 1

1 tablespoon vegetable glycerin

1 teaspoon aloe Vera gel

1 teaspoon rose water

8 drops of rose

4 drops of neroli

Blend 2

1 tablespoon shea butter

2 vitamin E capsules

1 teaspoon rosehip seed oil

Mix the above ingredients in a blender. Once blended, scoop out and add;

3 drops of lavender

10 drops of frankincense

5 drops of sandalwood

Blend 3

1 tablespoon melted beeswax

1 teaspoon melted coconut oil

1 teaspoon rosehip seed oil

6 drops of neroli

6 drops of jasmine

3 drops of rose

Allow the formula to solidify once all ingredients have been added.

Blend 4

1 tablespoons coconut oil

5 drops of geranium

5 drops of myrrh

5 drops of sandalwood

Cellulite

Cellulite is the buildup of fat, water and waste deposits under the skin, giving it a dimpled, lumpy appearance. It is a very frustrating condition and can be a major cause of misery for a lot of women. Thankfully essential oils can be a very effective remedy, when included with a healthy diet and exercise regime.

Essential oils for cellulite; Benzoin, Cedar wood, Cypress, Fennel, Geranium, Grapefruit, Juniper, Lemon, Mandarin, Orange, Rosemary, Thyme.

Carrier oils for cellulite; Sweet Almond Oil, Coconut Oil, Jojoba Oil.

Anti-Cellulite Plan (repeat daily):

Begin by dry brushing the entire body, using light upward strokes (always brush in the direction of the heart).

Have a warm to hot bath using the cellulite bath blends. Soak for 20 minutes. While soaking, pinch and deeply massage areas of cellulite to help break down fatty deposits.

Immediately after the bath (pores will be open),

apply a cellulite massage blend to the entire affected limb, for example, if you suffer from cellulite on the top of your legs, massage the entire leg and buttocks area. This will disperse the toxins and improve the flow of blood.

Drink 2 liters of water each day. This encourages the elimination of toxins. Do exercises that work specifically on the affected area. Use a cellulite body scrub and apply a cellulite body wrap 2-3 times per week.

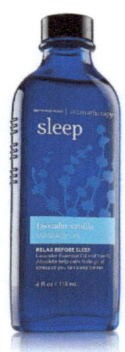

29. Massage Oils

Blend all ingredients together and mix thoroughly. Apply to the affected limb. When massaging, firmly grip the tissue, lifting it away from the muscles underneath. Using a kneading motion with your knuckles, rub the entire affected area as firmly as you can. Take care not to cause bruising but don't be afraid to massage firmly. Repeat daily.

Blend 1
2 tablespoons sweet almond oil
6 drops of benzoin
6 drops of rosemary
6 drops of cypress
6 drops of cedar wood

Blend 2
2 tablespoons coconut oil
6 drops of rosemary
6 drops of grapefruit
6 drops of fennel
6 drops of juniper

Blend 3
1 tablespoon sweet almond oil
1 tablespoon jojoba oil
6 drops of rosemary
6 drops of grapefruit
6 drops of thyme
6 drops of lemon

Blend 4

2 tablespoons sweet almond oil

6 drops of juniper

6 drops of mandarin

6 drops of geranium

6 drops of cedar wood

Blend 5

2 tablespoons coconut oil

10 drops of grapefruit

10 drops of rosemary

Blend 6

2 tablespoons jojoba oil

6 drops of thyme

6 drops of fennel

6 drops of juniper

6 drops of lemon

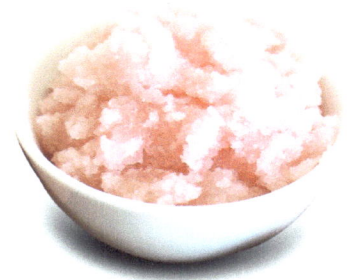

30. Body Scrubs

A body scrub can not only help lessen the appearance of cellulite, it also exfoliates the skin and improves circulation. This improved circulation will help to loosen up excess fluid and eliminate toxins at a quicker rate. Place all ingredients in a small bowl and mix thoroughly. Before a shower/bath, lather the scrub onto the affected area and massage into the skin using small, circular movements. Rinse off in the shower/bath and follow with a cellulite massage blend. Repeat 2-3 times per week.

Blend 1

½ cup ground coffee

½ cup brown sugar

2 tablespoons jojoba oil

10 drops of grapefruit

10 drops of rosemary

Blend 2

1 cup sea salt

2 tablespoons coconut oil

8 drops of fennel

8 drops of thyme

8 drops of thyme

8 drops of benzoin

8 drops of lemon

Blend 3

½ cup brown sugar

½ cup sea salt

1 tablespoon sweet almond oil

6 drops of grapefruit

6 drops of orange

6 drops of geranium

6 drops of juniper

Blend 4

1 cup ground oatmeal

2 tablespoons jojoba oil

5 drops of cedar wood

5 drops of cypress

5 drops of thyme

5 drops of mandarin

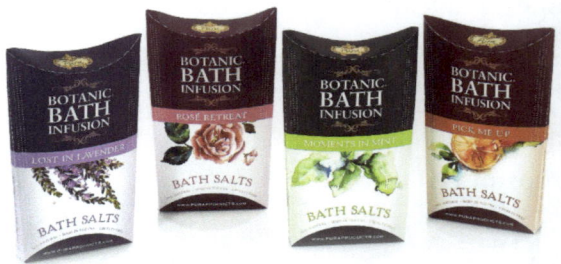

31. Bath Blends

A warm Epsom salt bath with essential oils is a great addition to your anti-cellulite regime. It helps to eliminate toxins from the body, while the essential oils absorb into the bloodstream, boosting circulation and stimulating lymph flow. Always add the Epsom salts before running the water, make sure the water is warm and not hot. Add the essential oils to the bath water and agitate the water to disperse the oils. While in the bath, firmly massage the affected area using circular knuckling movements. Soak for 20 minutes. Repeat daily. Drink 2 glasses of water after the bath.

Blend 1

2 cups Epsom salts

3 drops of juniper

3 drops of fennel

3 drops of cypress

3 drops of grapefruit

Blend 2

2 cups Epsom salts

5 drops of rosemary

5 drops of benzoin

3 drops of lemon

Blend 3

2 cups Epsom salts

15 drops of grapefruit

Blend 4

2 cups Epsom salts

5 drops of geranium

5 drops of orange

5 drops of lemon

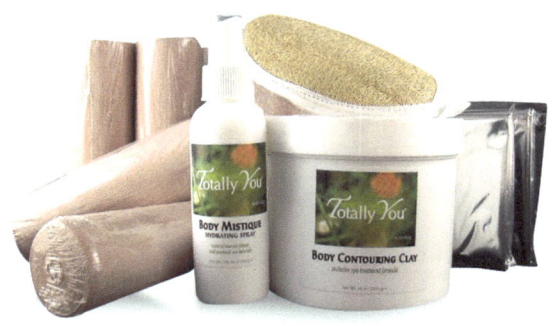

32. Body Wraps

Body wraps are designed to improve the texture and appearance of the skin by helping to rid the body of excess fluids and toxins. They are a fantastic way to help with cellulite and have many positive benefits including detoxification, skin tightening, skin softening and temporary inch loss.

To apply a body wrap;

· Blend all ingredients in a small bowl and mix thoroughly. Apply the formula over the affected area.

· You can cover the formula using either a roll of cling film or large rolls of elastic bandages (you will need 12-20 depending on the size of the area being treated).

· Begin by wrapping at the bottom of the area in question. Wrap tightly but not so tight as to cut off circulation.

· You can use a safety pin to hold the wraps in place but simply tucking the end of the bandage into the wrap itself will be sufficient.

· Do not expose any area of skin.

· Leave the wrap on for 30-45 minutes and during that time, drink 2 glasses of water.

· Depending on the ingredients used (for egg, clay, coffee or manuka honey) you may need to have a shower afterwards. For simple aromatherapy oil blends, a shower is not necessary.

Blend 1

5 tablespoons aloe Vera gel

15 drops of grapefruit

5 drops of cypress

Blend 2

½ cup extra virgin olive oil

5 drops of benzoin

5 drops of fennel

5 drops of lemon

5 drops of juniper

Blend 3

5 tablespoons manuka honey

5 tablespoons lemon juice

5 drops of grapefruit

5 drops of fennel

5 drops of juniper

Blend 4

½ cup coconut oil

4 tablespoons grapefruit juice

1 teaspoon baking soda

10 drops of rosemary

5 drops of lemon

5 drops of cypress

Blend 5

½ cup coconut oil

1 tablespoon lemon juice

10 drops of rosemary

10 drops of cedar wood

10 drops of geranium

Blend 6

½ cup ground coffee

½ cup sea salt

Juice of 1 lemon

5 drops of thyme

5 drops of cypress

5 drops of rosemary

Suggested daily cellulite regime using essential oils;

· Dry Brushing
· Warm bath
· Massage oils

Suggested cellulite regime - 2 to 3 times per week;

· Body scrub
· Warm bath
· Body wrap
· Massage oils

Chapped Lips

Because our lips do not contain oil glands, they are prone to dryness and chapping if not protected from the elements. Essential oils make for easy-to-make natural lip remedies.

Essential oils for chapped lips; Chamomile (Roman), Eucalyptus, Frankincense, Geranium, Neroli, Peppermint, Rose, Sandalwood, Tea Tree.

Carrier oils for chapped lips; Aloe Vera Gel (not a carrier oil but an effective treatment for chapped lips), Sweet Almond, Coconut, Rosehip.

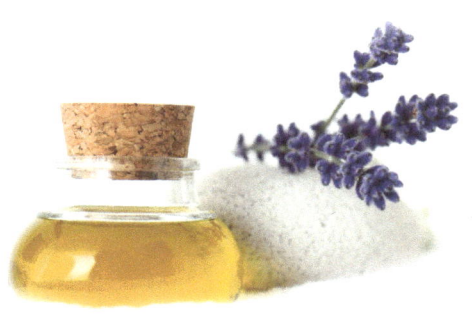

33. Massage Oils

Blend all ingredients together and mix thoroughly. Apply to lips. Leave to absorb, do not wash off. Repeat 2-3 times per day. The following recipes will make treatments for 1 day, apart from blend 4, this should last approximately 2-3 days.

Blend 1
1 teaspoon aloe Vera gel
2 drops of chamomile
2 drops of eucalyptus

Blend 2
1 teaspoon aloe Vera gel
3 drops of peppermint
1 drop of geranium

Blend 3
1 tablespoon extra-virgin olive oil
2 drops of lavender
2 drops of geranium

Blend 4
1 tablespoon beeswax pellets
1 tablespoon raw virgin coconut oil
2 vitamin E capsules
1 drop of frankincense
1 drops of lavender
1 drop of geranium
1 drop of peppermint

*melt the beeswax and coconut oil, add the essential oils and vitamin E capsule and leave to solidify.

Dilated Capillaries
Also known as broken capillaries or facial thread veins, this condition usually affects fair-skinned people and is the result of poor circulation or the loss of elasticity in capillary walls. Certain essential oils help to reduce vascularity, restore some elasticity to the blood vessels, and increase circulation.

Essential oils for dilated capillaries; Chamomile (Roman), Cypress, Geranium, Lemon, Neroli, Rose.

Carrier oils for dilated capillaries; Sweet Almond, Argan, Avocado, Borage Seed, Coconut, Evening Primrose, Wheat germ.

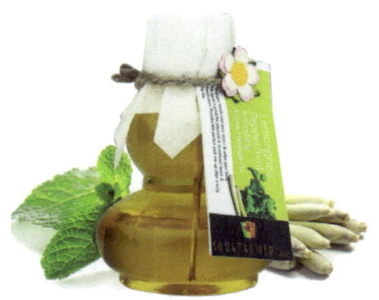

34. Massage Oils

Blend all ingredients together and mix thoroughly. Very gently massage the formula into the area in question. Leave to absorb into the skin, do not wash off. Repeat daily.

Blend 1
1 tablespoon Argan oil
1 teaspoon evening primrose oil
10 drops of chamomile
5 drops of rose

Blend 2
1 tablespoon coconut oil
5 drops of cypress
5 drops of neroli
5 drops of geranium

Blend 3
1 tablespoon sweet almond oil
8 drops of rosemary
7 drops of chamomile

Blend 4
1 tablespoon wheat germ oil
10ml borage seed oil
8 drops of cypress
5 drops of geranium
2 drops of neroli

Dry Skin

Dry skin is a common condition and occurs when the skin lacks either oil or moisture. It has the following characteristics;

· Small & tight pores
· Coarse and thin skin texture
· Uneven skin pigmentation
· Broken capillaries and premature ageing is common
· Patches of flaky skin may appear

When choosing essential oils for dry skin, choose oils that help to regenerate skin cells, reduce inflammation, balance the production of oil and help to reduce skin ageing.

Essential oils for dry skin include; Benzoin, Chamomile German, Frankincense, Geranium, Lavender, Myrrh, Neroli, Palmarosa, Patchouli, Rosemary, Rosewood, Sandalwood.

Carrier oils for dry skin include; Almond, Apricot Kernel, Avocado, Coconut, Evening Primrose, Jojoba, Macadamia, Peach Kernel.

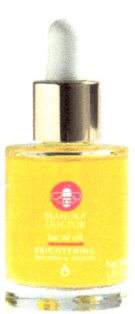

35. Facial Oils

Blend all the ingredients together and mix thoroughly. Apply the formula to a cleansed face and neck, and gently massage using small circular movements. Leave the oils to absorb into the skin cells, do not wash off. Carry out the treatment twice per day, once in the morning and again at night. At night, a facial oil can be substituted with a facial moisturizer (recipes below) if you prefer. The following recipes will yield enough for 1 treatment. Where coconut oil is used in these recipes, make sure to use Raw Virgin Coconut Oil as it is the best form of coconut oil to use for the skin. Melt it by placing an even tablespoon into a cup, place the cup into a saucepan of boiling water, and continue to boil the water on the heat until the coconut oil has melted. Never melt in the microwave.

Blend 1

1 tablespoon almond oil

8 drops of patchouli

8 drops of sandalwood

4 drops of myrrh

Blend 2

1 tablespoon jojoba oil

7 drops of Palmarosa

2 drops of rosemary

2 drops of sandalwood

2 drops of frankincense

Blend 3

1 tablespoon apricot kernel

4 drops of lavender

4 drops of chamomile

2 drops of geranium

2 drops of myrrh

Blend 4

1 tablespoon coconut oil

8 drops of frankincense

8 drops of myrrh

4 drops of neroli

2 drops of geranium

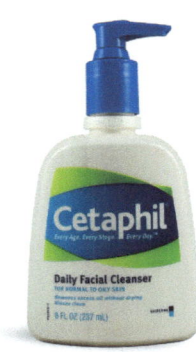

36. Facial Cleansers

Blend all ingredients together and mix thoroughly. Apply the formula to the face and neck, and massage into the skin using outward circular movements. Leave to absorb into the skin for 2 minutes. Gently remove all traces of oil, preferably using a wet muslin cloth soaked in warm water. A small, soft face towel can be used as an alternative. Repeat twice per day, once in the morning and again at night before applying a facial oil or moisturizer. The following recipes will yield enough for 1 treatment. Regarding coconut oil, please refer to 'Facial Oils' above for instructions on how to prepare. Where shea butter is used, melt it by placing an even tablespoon into a cup, place the cup in a saucepan of boiling water, and continue to boil the water on the heat until the shea butter has melted. Never melt in the microwave.

Blend 1

1 tablespoon coconut oil

9 drops of lavender

6 drops of geranium

Blend 2

1 tablespoon extra-virgin olive oil

6 drops of chamomile

6 drops of frankincense

Blend 3

1 tablespoon sweet almond oil

5 drops of Palmarosa

2 drops of rosemary

2 drops of lavender

Blend 4

1 tablespoon macadamia oil

6 drops of sandalwood

2 drops of patchouli

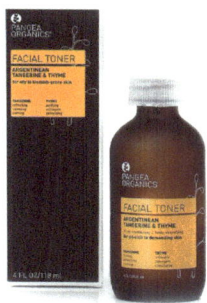

37. Facial Toners

Blend all ingredients in a glass bottle and shake well to combine. You can use a spray bottle if you wish but it is not necessary. Always add the hydrosol (flower water) first and then follow with the essential oils. Distilled water is a great alternative to hydrosols but always ensure you use distilled water (tap water may contain chemicals or bacteria). If you are using a spray bottle, hold it 3 to 4 inches away from the face, close your eyes and spray. Do not wipe off. If you are using a normal bottle, soak a cotton pad with the toner and gently pat all over the face and neck. Apply each time after cleansing, exfoliating or a face mask. The following recipes will yield enough for approximately 2 to 3 days.

Blend 1
50ml rose water
5 drops of lavender
5 drops of chamomile
5 drops of sandalwood

Blend 2
40ml lavender water
10ml distilled water
10 drops of geranium
10 drops of bergamot

Blend 3
1 teaspoon witch hazel
40ml aloe Vera juice
5 drops of Palmarosa
5 drops of rosewood
2 drops of chamomile

Blend 4
50ml rose water
15 drops of rosemary

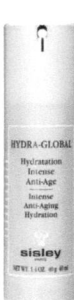

38. Facial Moisturizers

Blend all ingredients together and mix thoroughly. After cleansing and toning, apply the formula onto the face and neck, and massage into the skin, using small, gentle circular movements with the fingertips. If you are applying a day blend, allow the oils to absorb into the skin for 2 minutes before applying makeup. Repeat twice per day, once in the morning and again at night. A moisturizer may be substituted for a facial oil (recipes above) if you wish. The following recipes will yield enough for 1 - 2 treatments. Regarding coconut oil, please refer to 'Facial Oils' above for instructions on how to prepare.

Day Blend 1
1 tablespoon sweet almond oil
1 teaspoon jojoba oil
2 drops of lavender
2 drops of geranium
2 drops of Ylang Ylang

Day Blend 2
1 tablespoon coconut oil
6 drops of carrot seed
4 drops of myrrh
2 drops of frankincense
1 drop of lavender

Night Blend 1
1 tablespoon avocado oil
2 drops of rose
2 drops of neroli
2 drops of sandalwood

Night Blend 2
1 tablespoon wheat germ oil
1 teaspoon vitamin E oil (1 capsule)
4 drops of frankincense
4 drops of myrrh

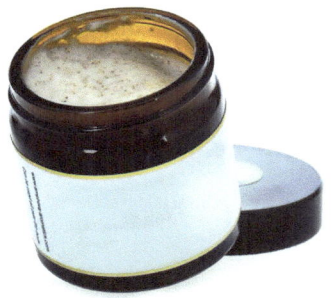

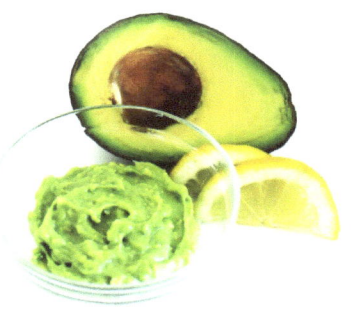

39. Facial Scrubs

Combine all ingredients in a small bowl, mix thoroughly and use immediately. Massage the blend gently into the skin as you would the facial cleanser. Leave on the skin for 2 minutes and wash off with warm water. Carry out this treatment once per week. The following recipes will yield enough for 1 treatment. Regarding coconut oil, please refer to 'Facial Oils' above for instructions on how to prepare.

Blend 1
1 cup of ground oatmeal
4 tablespoons of avocado oil
8 drops of patchouli
4 drops of Ylang Ylang
4 drops of chamomile

Blend 2
2 large tablespoons of manuka honey
½ cup of brown sugar
1 tablespoon of extra virgin olive oil
2 drops of geranium
2 drops of bergamot
1 drop of lavender

40. Facial Masks

Blend all ingredients in a small bowl, mix thoroughly and use immediately. Apply the formula with either a mask brush or clean fingers, after the skin has been cleansed. Leave on for 15 to 20 minutes and wash off with warm water. Pat dry the face, follow with a toner and moisturizer or facial oil. Apply a face mask once every week. The following recipes will yield enough for 1 treatment.

Blend 1
1 ripe avocado (mashed)
1 tablespoon of coconut oil
8 drops of frankincense
4 drops of myrrh
2 drops of chamomile

Blend 2
2 tablespoons of manuka honey
4 drops of Ylang Ylang
2 drops of geranium
2 drops of sandalwood

Blend 3
3 tablespoons of aloe Vera gel
½ teaspoon of jojoba oil
6 drops of lavender
2 drops of Palmarosa
2 drops of rosemary

Blend 4
2 tablespoons of unflavored yogurt
6 drops of neroli
4 drops of chamomile

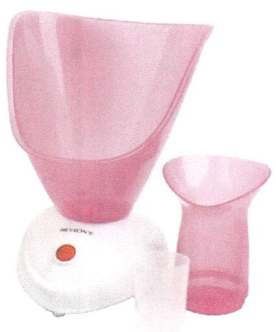

41. Facial Sauna

Fill a large bowl with boiling water, add the chosen essential oils, place a towel around your head and lean towards the water (closing off the sides with the towel). The steam can burn your skin so hold your head as close as is comfortable. Close eyes and inhale deeply for 7 - 10 minutes.

Blend 1
1 large bowl of boiling water
8 drops of sandalwood

Blend 2
1 large bowl of boiling water
3 drops of lavender
3 drops of geranium
2 drops of frankincense

Hair Care
Essential oils can work wonders for the hair, whether you want to treat a dry, flaky scalp, stimulate hair growth, strengthen hair or improve the condition. Choose from one of the following categories below and follow the recipes regularly for healthy, shiny hair.

Dandruff
Dandruff is a common dry scalp condition which causes flaking of the scalp and itching. It can be a very embarrassing and frustrating condition for some people but thankfully essential oils are a very effective way to treat and alleviate the problem.

Essential oils for dandruff; Basil, Cypress, Lavender, Lemon, Peppermint, Rosemary, Tea Tree, Thyme.

Carrier oils for dandruff; Borage Seed, Coconut, Evening Primrose, Jojoba.

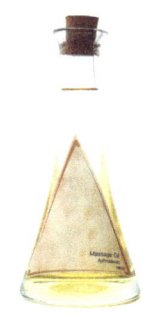

42. Massage Oils

Blend all ingredients together and mix thoroughly. Pour a small amount into the palm of your hand and gently rub both hands together to evenly spread the formula. Massage it into the scalp, starting at the top of the forehead. Continue to apply the blend to the entire scalp until the oils have been used up. For 5 minutes, gently massage the scalp using the pads of the fingers in small, circular movements. Keep the blend on overnight or for as long as you can. Rinse and condition the hair as normal (add several drops of the same essential oils to your shampoo to boost results). Repeat 2-3 times per week. The following recipes will make 1 treatment.

Blend 1

1 tablespoon jojoba oil

1 tablespoon evening primrose oil

5 drops of rosemary

5 drops of lavender

5 drops of peppermint

Blend 2

2 tablespoons coconut oil

15 drops of tea tree

Blend 3

2 tablespoons jojoba oil

6 drops of basil

4 drops of lemon

3 drops of rosemary

2 drops of thyme

Blend 4

2 tablespoons macadamia oil

10 drops of tea tree

5 drops of rosemary

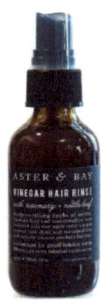

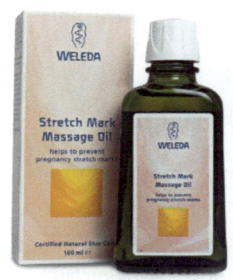

43. Hair Rinse

Blend all ingredients together and mix thoroughly. Massage into your scalp after shampooing/rinsing your hair. Leave for 5 minutes and rinse. Condition and style as normal. Repeat 2-3 times per week. The following recipes will make 1 treatment.

Blend 1
½ cup apple cider vinegar
10 drops of peppermint
5 drops of tea tree
5 drops of lavender

Blend 2
½ cup witch hazel
10 drops of tea tree
10 drops of rosemary

Dry, Damaged or Frizzy Hair
Dry hair is caused by the underproduction of oil glands in the scalp which results in the hair becoming dry, brittle and tangled. It can be further aggravated by the use of bleaching, tinting and regular hair coloring. Regular treatments using essential oils can nourish the scalp, rebalance oil production and condition and soften the hair.

Essential oils for dry, damaged or frizzy hair;
Geranium, Lavender, Palmarosa, Rosemary, Sandalwood.

Carrier oils for dry, damaged or frizzy hair;
Coconut, Jojoba, Macadamia, Olive, Peach Kernel.

44. Massage Oils

Blend all ingredients together and mix thoroughly. Pour a small amount into the palm of your hands and massage it into the scalp (add more oil if your hair is longer or thicker). Apply the remaining formula throughout the hair, making sure to cover the ends. Gently massage the scalp using small, circular movements for about 5 minutes. Leave on for several hours or overnight if you can (remember to protect your bed sheets). Rinse the treatment out thoroughly and condition your hair as normal. Repeat 2-3 times per week for the best results. Each of the following recipes carries out 1 treatment.

Blend 1
3 tablespoons jojoba oil
10 drops of lavender
5 drops of sandalwood

Blend 2
2 tablespoons olive oil
5 drops of sandalwood
5 drops of Palmarosa
5 drops of lavender
5 drops of rosemary
5 drops of geranium

Blend 3
3 tablespoons macadamia oil
10 drops of sandalwood
10 drops of lavender
5 drops of rosemary

Blend 4
2 tablespoons coconut oil
25 drops of lavender

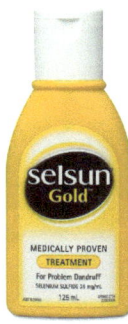

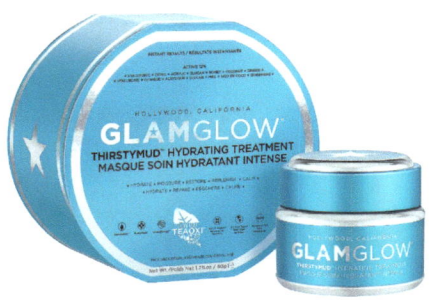

45. Treatment Shampoo

Blend all ingredients together in a bowl and mix thoroughly. Apply to wet hair and massage into the scalp and hair. You may need to include more base shampoo depending on the length and thickness of your hair. The following formulas are for 1 treatment on medium length hair.

Blend 1
2 tablespoons unscented natural shampoo
1 vitamin E capsules
1 teaspoon jojoba oil
5 drops of sandalwood
5 drops of geranium

Blend 2
2 tablespoons unscented natural shampoo
1 teaspoon macadamia oil
5 drops of lavender
5 drops of Palmarosa

46. Treatment Masks

Adding a mask treatment to your healthy hair regime can really boost results by helping to further condition, nourish and improve the texture of hair. Blend all ingredients in a small bowl and mix thoroughly. Apply to damp, clean hair. Divide the hair into section and massage the mask into the hair and scalp, paying particular attention to the ends. Leave on for 1 hour and thoroughly rinse and condition hair as normal. Repeat twice per week. Each of the following recipes are for 1 treatment on medium length hair.

Blend 1
2 tablespoons coconut milk
1 tablespoon raw, unprocessed honey
2 tablespoons extra virgin olive oil
10 drops of lavender
5 drops of sandalwood

Blend 2
½ ripe avocado (mashed)
1 tablespoon jojoba oil
1 tablespoon macadamia oil
5 drops of rosemary
5 drops of Palmarosa
5 drops of geranium

Hair Lice
Lice are parasites that infest the hair and must be dealt with immediately as they can spread by direct contact. Compared to traditional pharmaceutical treatments, essential oils are a non-toxic, safe alternative for eliminating head lice as they can effectively kill lice and their eggs.

Essential oils for head lice; Eucalyptus, Geranium, Lavender, Lavender, Lemon, Rosemary, Tea Tree, Thyme.

Carrier oils for head lice; Sweet Almond, Coconut, Evening Primrose, Grape seed, Jojoba.

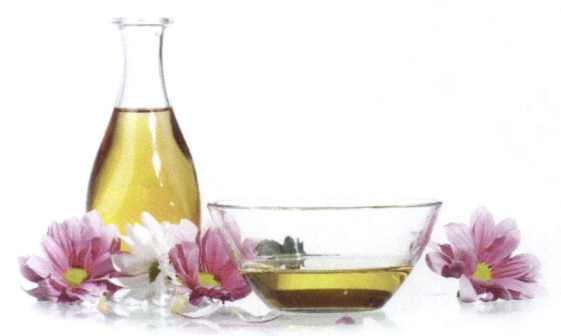

47. Massage Oils

Blend all ingredients together and mix thoroughly. Wash, (shampoo with added drops of tea tree will boost results), towel dry and meticulously comb the hair. Vigorously massage the formula into the scalp, ensuring that the entire scalp is covered. Leave the treatment on for 2-3 hours and rinse. Repeat each night until the lice have been eliminated. The following recipes will make 1 treatment.

Blend 1
3 tablespoons coconut oil
15 drops of tea tree
10 drops of lavender
5 drops of rosemary

Blend 2
3 tablespoons jojoba oil
10 drops of rosemary
10 drops of geranium
10 drops of lavender

Blend 3
3 tablespoons grape seed oil
10 drops of eucalyptus
10 drops of rosemary
5 drops of lemon
5 drops of lavender

Blend 4
3 tablespoons coconut oil
10 drops of lemon
10 drops of tea tree
10 drops of thyme

Hair Loss & Regrowth

The most important factor to consider when treating any kind of hair loss is a healthy scalp. Massaging the scalp regularly with certain essential oils stimulates the blood vessels of the scalp to send vital nutrients and oxygen to the hair follicles at a faster rate. Over time, this encourages growth and improves the condition and texture of hair.

Essential oils for hair loss & regrowth; Cedar wood, Chamomile (Roman), Clary Sage, Cypress, Lavender, Lemon, Rosemary, Thyme.

Carrier oils for hair loss & regrowth; Coconut, Evening Primrose, Grape seed, Jojoba.

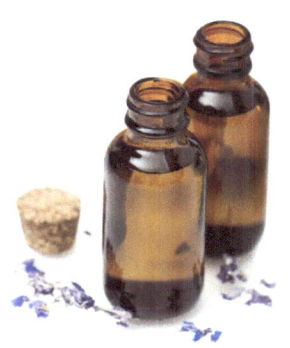

48. Massage Oils

Blend all ingredients together and mix thoroughly. Pour a small amount into the palm of your hand and gently rub both hands together to evenly spread the formula. Massage it into the scalp, starting at the top of the forehead. Continue to apply the blend to the entire scalp until the oils have been used up. For 5 minutes, gently massage the scalp using the pads of the fingers in small, circular movements. Keep the blend on overnight or for as long as you can. Rinse and condition the hair as normal (add several drops of the same essential oils to your shampoo to boost results). Repeat 2-3 times per week. The following recipes will make 1 treatment.

Blend 1
2 tablespoons grape seed
1 teaspoon jojoba oil
5 drops of lavender
5 drops of thyme
5 drops of rosemary

Blend 2
2 tablespoons jojoba
8 drops of rosemary
7 drops of thyme

Blend 3
1 tablespoon jojoba oil
1 tablespoon macadamia oil
5 drops of thyme
5 drops of cedar wood
5 drops of clary sage

Blend 4
1 tablespoon coconut oil
1 tablespoon evening primrose oil
6 drops of rosemary
4 drops of lavender
2 drops of cypress
2 drops of chamomile

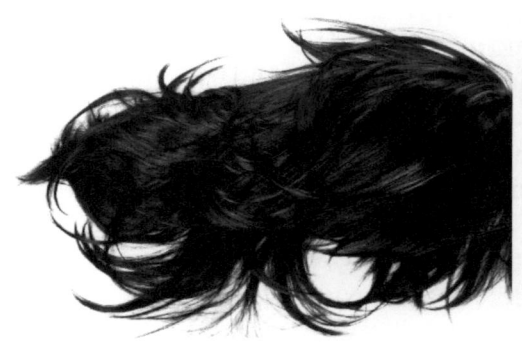

Oily Hair

Oily hair is the result of the overproduction of oil glands in the scalp. Hair is characteristically limp and lifeless, and can look greasy. Shampoo with harsh chemicals and detergents can often worsen the problem as they stimulate excess oil production, so including more natural products in your hair care regime is recommended.

Essential oils for oily hair; Cypress, Grapefruit, Juniper Berry, Lavender, Lemon, Peppermint, Rosemary.

Carrier oils for oily hair; Sweet Almond, Coconut, Grape seed, Jojoba.

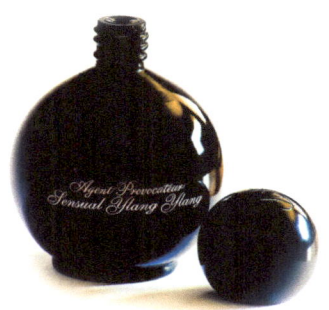

Blend 4
2 tablespoons sweet almond oil
10 drops of cypress
10 drops of rosemary
5 drops of grapefruit

49. Massage Oils

Blend all ingredients together and mix thoroughly. Pour a small amount into the palm of your
hands and massage it into the scalp (add more
oil if your hair is longer or thicker). Apply the
remaining formula throughout the hair, making
sure to cover the ends. Gently massage the scalp
using small, circular movements for about 5 minutes. Leave on for several hours or overnight if
you can (remember to protect your bed sheets).
Rinse the treatment out thoroughly and condition your hair as normal. Repeat 2-3 times per
week for the best results. Each of the following
recipes carries out 1 treatment.

Blend 1
2 tablespoons jojoba oil
10 drops of cypress
5 drops of lemon
5 drops of lavender
5 drops of rosemary

Blend 2
2 tablespoons grape seed oil
5 drops of peppermint
5 drops of lavender
5 drops of cypress
5 drops of juniper berry
5 drops of lemon

Blend 3
2 tablespoons coconut oil
10 drops of lemon
10 drops of lavender
5 drops of peppermint

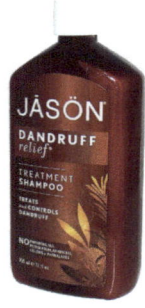

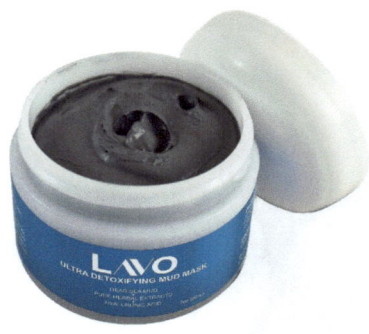

50. Treatment Shampoo

Blend all ingredients together in a bowl and mix thoroughly. Apply to wet hair and massage into the scalp and hair. You may need to include more base shampoo depending on the length and thickness of your hair. The following formulas are for 1 treatment on medium length hair.

Blend 1
1 tablespoon unscented natural shampoo
1 teaspoon apple cider vinegar
6 drops of lemon
4 drops of cypress

Blend 2
1 tablespoon unscented natural shampoo
1 tablespoon coconut milk
4 drops of rosemary
4 drops of peppermint
2 drops of juniper berry

51. Treatment Masks

Adding a mask treatment to your healthy hair regime can really boost results by helping to further condition, nourish and improve the texture of hair. Blend all ingredients in a small bowl and mix thoroughly. Apply to damp, clean hair. Divide the hair into section and massage the mask into the hair and scalp, paying particular attention to the ends. Leave on for 1 hour and thoroughly rinse and condition hair as normal. Repeat twice per week. Each of the following recipes is for 1 treatment on medium length hair.

Blend 1
1 tablespoon raw unprocessed honey
Juice from ½ lemon
1 teaspoon jojoba oil
10 drops of rosemary
4 drops of lavender

Blend 2
1 tablespoon baking soda
1 tbsp. apple cider vinegar
5 drops of lemon
5 drops of peppermint
5 drops of cypress

conclusion

One of the best things about essential oils is the fact that they don't require you to be an aroma therapist in order to benefit from them. Anyone can use them and some come when they are already pre-blended so you don't have to worry about how to go about the process of blending them. What is required of you is simply putting them in a burner or rubbing them on the various pulse joints.

You don't need to have complicated issues to require essential oils. You can use them for something as simple as a burn. Pour cold water on it and use the recommended essential oil such as a mixture of lavender oil and sweet almond oil.

More people are going back to the traditional ways of treatments and preferring natural remedies. This is why the number of people resorting to using essential oils is rising because they can offer greater therapeutic benefits without the worry of the harmful side effects. Try out the essential oils and experience the benefits first hand.

Did You Like Aromatherapy and Essential Oils?

Before you go, we'd like to say "thank you" for purchasing our book. So a big thanks for downloading this book and reading all the way to the end. Now we'd like to ask for a *small* favor. Could you please take a minute or two and leave a review for this book on Amazon

This feedback will help us continue to write the kind of Kindle books that help you get results. And if you loved it, then please let me know

Click here to leave a review for this book on Amazon!

Check Out My Other Books

Below you'll find some of my other popular books that are popular on Amazon and Kindle as well. Simply click on the links below to check them out. Alternatively, you can visit my author page on Amazon to see other work done by me.

www.amazon.com/author/jjlewis

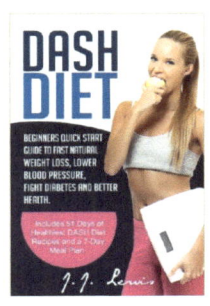 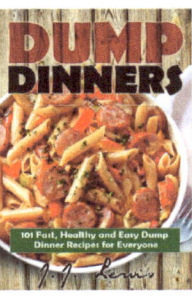 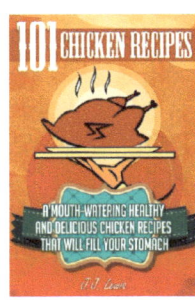 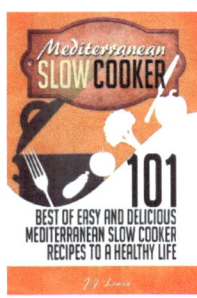 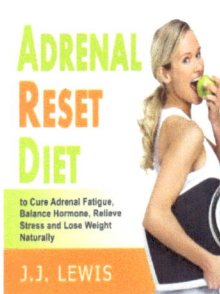

Dash Diet: Beginners Quick Start Guide to Fast Natural Weight Loss, Lower Blood

Dump Dinners: 101 Fast, Healthy and Easy Dump Dinner Recipes for Everyone

Adrenal Reset Diet: 51 Days of Powerful Adrenal Diet Recipes to Cure Adrenal Fatigue, Balance Hormone, Relieve Stress and Lose Weight Naturally

Mediterranean Slow Cooker: 101 Best of Easy and Delicious Mediterranean Slow Cooker Recipes to a Healthy Life

101 Chicken Recipes: A Mouth-Watering Healthy and Delicious Chicken Recipes that will fill your Stomach

Paleo Slow Cooker: 101 Quick and Easy Paleo Recipes for Healthy Life and Weight

101 Pork Chop Recipes: Extraordinary and Delicious Pork Chop Recipes for Everyday Meals

101 Vegetarian Recipes: Top Vegan Diet Recipes to Live a Healthy Lifestyle

Ketogenic Diet: 101 Days of Ketogenic Diet, Low Carb Recipes for Maximum Weight Loss Benefits

Pressure Cooker Recipes: 101 Mouthwatering, Delicious, Easy and Healthy Pressure Cooker Recipes for Breakfast, Lunch, Dinner in 30 Minutes or Less!

Vegan Cookbook: Vegan Diet for Beginners to a Healthy Everyday Life (Vegan Appetizers and Soups Series)

Paleo Diet: 101 Days of Easy Paleo Diet Recipes Made for Beginners to Maximize Weight Loss

Paleo Diet for Kids: A Fun Pack of 101 Flavorful and Energy-Boosting Paleo Recipes Best In Shaping Healthier, Stronger and Happier Paleo-Nourished Kids

Slow Cooker Recipes: The Best of 101 Nutritious and Delicious Healthy Slow-Cooking Recipes for your Crock Pot

The Juice Cleanse: 101 Healthy Juicing Recipes for Weight Loss

Fast Metabolism Diet Recipes: 101 Best of Metabolism Boosting Recipes to Lose Weight Fast
Low Fat Recipes: 101 Incredible Quick & Easy Recipes for a Low Fat Diet
Gluten Free Diet: 101 Delectable and Healthy Gluten-Free Recipes for better life-style
Diabetes Diet: 101 Healthy Diabetes Recipes to Reverse Diabetes Forever and Enjoy Healthy Living for Life
Wheat Belly Diet: 101 Days of Grain Free Recipes for an Optimum Belly Diet and Weight Loss

If the links do not work, for whatever reason, you can simply search for these titles on the Amazon website to find them.

Want more Bestseller Cook Books for **FREE?**

Join my **V.I.P** Reading List where I give away Healthy and Delicious Recipes **FOR FREE!**

Yes, you heard me right! COMPLETELY FREE to everyone just for being a loyal reader of mine!

JOIN FREE BY CLICKING HERE!

www.ingramcontent.com/pod-product-compliance
Lightning Source LLC
Chambersburg PA
CBHW041503280526
45792CB00004B/1117